Goodbye, House
The Emotional Journey

Marilyn Moldowan

Copyright © 2017 Marilyn Moldowan

All rights reserved. No part of this book may be reproduced or transmitted in any form or by any means without written permission of the publisher, except in the case of brief quotations embodied in critical articles and reviews.

This material has been written and published solely for educational purposes. The author and the publisher shall have neither liability nor responsibility to any person or entity with respect to any loss, damage, or injury caused or alleged to be caused directly or indirectly by the information contained in this book.

Statements made and opinions expressed in this publication are those of the author and do not necessarily reflect the views of the publisher or indicate an endorsement by the publisher.

Goodbye House

We take our houses for granted sometimes. The roof over our heads keeps us safe from the elements, the walls around us demarcate the space in which we live, and the central heat, air conditioning, electricity and running water are the creature comforts that we have come to expect in our part of the world. We are physically safe in our houses.

But when does the house become a home? Is there one thing that defines the feeling that you are "home"? It is more than the four walls and the ceiling. Why is it so hard for us to say good bye to a house?

Circumstances are different for all of us when we move, but the one constant is that everyone has some sort of emotional response, there is a unique emotional journey and experience. This is the one common thread that fascinated me. I dug a little deeper: conversation with people at different stages of moving from their homes created more questions. Why do we have such an attachment to plaster, wood and carpet? When does that connection begin? How do people move away from a home they've been in, sometimes for decades? These conversations created more questions than they answered.

Research around the adult children of seniors, seniors themselves and the process of moving and selling the family home, provided no concrete answers. The decision making that occurs was as individual as the family unit. The responses and feelings after the home had been sold, range widely. Some families were matter of fact and said "wow, I'm so glad that is done", without much emotional fanfare at all. These families saw the sale as just that, a sale, and a necessary part of the way things had to be. At the far other send of the spectrum are the families whose response was more like a grieving and the angst of the decision was palpable. In the event of a crisis where the transition and sale happened quickly, there was almost a feeling of "soul" trauma.

The emotional journey intrigues me.

In the book, "Carry Me Out Toes First", I try to define what a home really means: "…there is a place where we house our bodies, where we keep our treasures, where we eat, sleep and love, where we raise our families and welcome our grandchildren. We take a tiny speck of space, carve it gently out of the universe, and we call this place home…"

More and more adult children are finding that their parents are requiring increasingly more support in order for them to stay in their own homes. Any attempt at a conversation could be absolutely shut down by the parent, resisted or stymied, or simply brushed off as a "yes, I know, but now is not the time for me to move". At other times, it can be very poignant to realize that there may not be a choice in the matter. However, every family is different, their dynamics are different and life circumstances are different. What is the same in every case, however, is the fact that there is grieving and an incredible amount of personal energy that any "move" takes out of everyone involved.

This book is meant to be a guide in how to better navigate that process.

It is a process that can take years, actually. The information provided here can be the bridge between the business of moving and the wisdom of home. Almost without exception, once the heart is wrapped around the need or the desire for a move, the actual physical move, the business part, the logical part, is much easier. All the logic in the world cannot make someone do anything that they are not ready to do. The heart will not follow the head, but the head will follow the heart. Once the heart says "yes" to a move, then all the logic in the world will not convince someone otherwise. Through examples, stories and tangible suggestions, this book will identify some ways to bridge the "business" part of the move with the wisdom of "home".

Let's begin, then, with outlining some of the behaviours and decisions that may make it easier to say goodbye to your house. Sometimes a story better illustrates the point and those are included as well.

Choose to Stay

The very first step in the process of emotionally detaching might quite simply be to just stay put. Although this seems counter-intuitive, there are many powerful reasons for this choice. Especially in a situation where a family member is adamant that there is no way in hell they are moving, there needs to be an honoring of that decision. Just because we don't like someone's decision does not make that person incompetent. Often, the definition of competency includes the ability to manage finances, taking care of the bills, keeping the home maintained and the attention to their own personal needs. If the person thinks that they are doing all this quite well on their own, they will tell you to go whistle, thank you very much!

There may be other factors besides an intense pride at being able to still live independently. In fact, here is dignity associated with the decision to live "at risk" and there are little victories every day when someone chooses to go this route. They are beating the odds and doing it their way. (Thank you, Frank Sinatra!)

Frieda is a widow in her eighties who openly admits that she has stayed in her home for as long as she has because it gives her a purpose. The tasks of maintaining an old house on a quarter acre lot is never ending and it is "frustrating" for her to sometimes not get everything done that she wants to. However, Frieda says that if she sold her house she would lose her personality. She takes pride in being able to talk knowledgably with the repair people that she hires, and she knows when she is not being treated fairly. The amount of yard she takes care of keeps her active and limber. She does her own snow shoveling in the winter in 15 minute segments, a little at a time, and goes back inside the house to warm up or get a drink then goes out again.

Frieda is a delight to talk with, a woman with sharp intellect and deprecating humour. Her one lament is that she has a lack of trust. It used to be, she explains, that you could open your door to anyone. If someone knocked, there was a good reason, but she never opens the door these days to anyone who she is not expecting. In fact, it really gets her "Irish up" when a salesperson tries to talk her into something she does not want and he quickly finds out that Frieda is nobody's fool.

She has a mountain view and is a block from the river. There is nature around her and she is proud of the location of her home. Sitting in her tranquil backyard, you can't tell that you are in the middle of a large city. Frieda's address, too, means something to her as it is distinguished and is a symbol of the life that she and her husband created together. She savours those memories, and I can see her eyes turn inward as she describes those days.

Needless to say, she's not going anywhere. Her emotional journey was her intense pride and feeling of independence.

In another province, far away, a different circumstance played out.

Dora was feeling very vulnerable and alone after her husband passed away. Even though her children visited as often as they could in the year after his passing, they all had jobs in other cities and lived several hours away. the year after his passing, they all had jobs in other cities and lived several hours away. Dora's husband was the fix-it guy, and he the year after his passing, they all had jobs in other cities and lived several hours away. the year after his passing, they all had jobs in other cities and lived several hours away. Dora's husband was the fix-it guy, and he maintained the house very well. She never worried about a leaky tap or broken window, as Dan would always take care of it. He had most recently arranged to have the shingles replaced and a new furnace installed. When he was no longer able to take care of the yard, Dan arranged for a lawn care and snow removal company.

Dan was also the driver in the house. Dora never did get her driver's license because she felt as though she never had to. Living in the city, she walked for groceries to the nearby supermarket and, if there were larger items to be purchased, Dan was always happy to do the "hauling". Any other appointments were the same: Dan enjoyed the driving.

Dora did not want to move from the house, but she was finding the loneliness nearly unbearable and craved another human voice. Repairs were beginning to crop up, and, although she tried her best to find a reputable company, she felt sometimes that the charges were just a little on the high side. Dora took taxi's in the winter but just hated to spend the money to go the ten blocks to the shopping center, a distance that she easily walked in the summer.

During a phone call with one of her daughters, Dora became emotional and shared all the reasons why it was becoming more difficult to stay. As luck would have it, the company Lisa worked for was in transition. Lisa was looking for other opportunities and Mother and daughter came up with a plan. It worked beautifully for the entire family.

Lisa found a solid job in the city where Dora lived, and moved back into the home. Dora had company, someone to help with the increasing maintenance and, of course, Lisa had a car! In return for a place to live, Lisa bought the groceries for the house, drove her Mom to appointments and gave her Mom peace of mind by simply being close by.

The rest of the family also saw the gift in this arrangement. They relaxed, knowing that their Mom was no longer alone.

This family found a solution to the emotional journey that they were all on. Eventually, they will say "Goodbye, House", but for now their Mom has a chance to live life the way she wants to, and the family has become an even more cohesive unit.

Now, granted, this type of arrangement may not work for every family, but for these people, the stars aligned to create a better emotional experience for all concerned.

Begin to Declutter

Part of the emotional preparation involves the clearing out of the items in your home that no longer really serve any useful purpose. I recommend looking at the things that have no emotional charge on them, the ones that are simply neutral items.

In her book, "The Art of Discarding" by Nagisa Tatsumi, the author indicates that so much of what we choose to keep are, as she labels them, "nuisance items". Pens that don't work, cups with a crack in them, a blouse with a small stain, old business cards, or pretty much anything in that kitchen junk drawer can be discarded.

Begin with the habit of taking two bags out for every one that you bring in. For instance, one bag of groceries brought into the house means that by the end of that day you have two bags by the back door ready to be removed from the home. The two bags can be old papers or magazines for recycling, old clothes to be given away or simply two bags of plain old garbage.

There is great advantage, too, in starting to

use up the stockpiles of paper goods, canned food and spices. The clearing out of the kitchen cabinets will provide hours of entertainment, and many people laugh at what they have chosen to keep stored away. Please stay away from bulk-buying anything else. Really, how dirty IS your bum that you need all that toilet paper?

One family decided to completely empty out the basement of the family home over the course of a summer. About a year after their Dad passed away, the Mom was looking for suggestions from the adult children on how she could slowly start the downsize process for herself, since she no longer had her husband to discuss this with. She went into the basement to do laundry but the last time anyone else used the bedroom or the television down there was at the Father's funeral. There were items stored in every nook and cranny that had layers of dust on them from years on non-use : decades old children's toys, jars and lids from the canning she used to do, and lamps, small side tables and torn sheets and towels. The list went on and on.

They started by removing any of the furniture that could be used by other family members. A grandchild was going to college and had an apartment that needed furniture. Other items were sold at a garage sale, some were "free if you could carry it away" and the remainder of items were simply discarded. It was done over the course of a few weeks and the Mother had fabulous support from all family members. The thing she really liked about the entire process of preparation for an eventual house sale, is that she got to choose and she got a say in "what went where". More recently, her own health is declining. She simply loves the fact that the basement will not be an area of concern for her family when she decides to sell her home. It is like a great weight lifted from her shoulders.

Re-purpose and Re-love

As you begin to go through the stuff that is just stuff, the neutral items, what you will find is that it does become easier to place something into the trash bag or into recycling. The mindset of purging that which no longer serves you, feels very good once you get it started.

Then there is an "oops". You come across something that does have some meaning and even though it really has no use, there is emotion attached to it. I'm not talking about the dining room table, chairs and hutch that have been passed down from your mother's mother. I'm thinking about the emotion that is experienced in finding the hammer that your Father used for everything from hanging pictures to building the fence and loosening bolts while rebuilding the car engine. This jolt of memory can catch you off guard. It's those items that you have forgotten about, and when they are in your hands again, they can unleash memories and sometimes, tears.

This is good. I call it "feasting on your life". It is a chance to re-live and feel once again, the presence of that event. This emotion is part of the journey of detachment. It is meant to rehonor and feel again the life that was once in the home as the memory can still tug at your heart. It will be those items that are tucked away, those items that you've forgotten about, that will create this type of precious remembering.

With every family gathering, try to re-purpose an item or two. Maybe the hammer that you found tucked away means a lot to a daughter because it was the one used when Dad built her dollhouse decades ago. An old hand held mirror that Grandma used to check her makeup before she married Grandpa could be passed on to the next lady in the family who is planning to become a wife. The small cabinet beside Uncle's bed may be the perfect size and height for a small child's book case. Re-love and re-purpose a little at a time, over the course of many months, or even years. As the cabinets and bookcases slowly empty out, give them away so that they are not accessible.

One family actually had family dinners with the idea that at the end of the evening, when the kitchen was clean and the china was washed up, that pieces of the dinnerware and crystal would be lovingly taken by each member of the family.

There is a couple who live in an apartment complex, and they have a storage locker in the basement of the building. Over the course of a couple weeks, they emptied all the contents of the storage locker and now have that same locker rented out to another resident in the building. No, the couple didn't move the contents to their suite….they recycled, repurposed and discarded. And they have begun to do the same with one of the bedrooms in their apartment. Their example is proof that it all does not have to happen at once.

Document the Good Memories

The emotional journey can sometimes be tough, and every situation is a little different. Saying good bye means that the special moments cannot be re-lived. Your home is not just an inanimate structure where you have found shelter from the winter storms or rested after a long day at work. The fear of forgetting the precious moments of fun and hearty laughter could be very real, or maybe there's a concern about disconnecting from the love that was felt in the home.

An entry in a recent blog with the website "DesignSponge" delves into those good memories. This is an excerpt from that writing:

"…In some homes, the soul of the space has been lovingly crafted over time. The memories we make there, bit by bit, laugh by laugh, with some heartache thrown in for good measure, make it inconceivable to ever abandon the house itself. We say that it's the memories and people that make a home, not the things in it or the structure itself, yet when we're forced to leave a treasured home behind, it doesn't merely tug at the heart strings-it damn near severs them.

I've left old apartments behind before, and while I was sad to leave certain aspects….I never anticipated the mourning that ensued when we began the process of selling my parent's home…

I never truly lived in this home like my younger brother and sister did. Construction completed when I was in college, and throughout my four years just two hours away I'd never spent more than a month or two there at a time. This was never, in a sense of living, my home.

But in the sense of SOUL, this was my 'home' through and through. We lived in this house. Friends always felt welcome like it was their home, and treated it as such. A whirlwind of moments from those ten years would reveal late nights musing over a favourite song, wine in hand, or Christmas mornings, when my Dad would play the same song every year as we gathered around the tree to open gifts (Johnny Mathis' "Sleigh Ride"), the smell of Mom's egg strata in the oven; or the New Year's Day when we all jumped into the hot tub in our pyjamas.

The memories created there took on more profound meaning than ever before after my Dad was diagnosed with cancer. We clung to each other and to our constant-the house. The house didn't let us down, it pulled us in and made us feel safe when we were so scared we couldn't think straight. It reverberated the sound of Dad's favourite Van Morrison songs. It wore the tread of visitors trickling in and out to spend time with us. It echoed the crying-it amplified the laughter. It kept bending and creasing, like a giant old sweatshirt, to be exactly what we needed when we didn't even know WHAT we needed.

And it continued to wrap us in its walls. Even after Dad passed away. The memories were suddenly immortalized. Our home was unconditional and selfless. A steadfast confidant.

So what is it that makes us mourn the loss of a structure? It's not the great architecture, or the way the light pours in through the windows in the morning. It's almost as if leaving a home rich in such a lived-in history causes our memories to spill out everywhere, and we feel like we've spun out of orbit, scrambling to collect them.

It is possible to grieve the passing of a home, too."

Document your memories. Write them down. Create a journal. Take those pictures. Salvage the old ones.

Say Goodbye to Each Room

Joshua Green is a moving industry professional who makes this suggestion as part of the emotional journey of saying goodbye. Photos and stories alone are not sufficient for some families, and a more genuine goodbye can be experienced by going to the next level. Gather up the family, go through each room of the house and let everyone bid their own special farewell by telling an interesting story that happened there and reminiscing about a happy and fun memory related to that particular room. A video camera can create a "living scrapbook of memories to keep the past alive." After each family member has taken their proper goodbyes, leave the room together as a unit and close the door behind you as a symbolic gesture of moving on. Go to the next room and do it all over again. If there are grandchildren, it will enable them to prepare mentally and accept the upcoming change, but it can also serve as an indicator for the level of happiness while they were visiting their Grandparents in that house.

Take Something With You

Even though it sounds unusual, take a meaningful piece of your house with you to your new home. This isn't about the items that are going with you anyway, but rather, taking a precious souvenir that means something only to you. The object is charged with a concentrated value of meaningfulness that only you understand. Remove the door handle on the favourite room of the house or the lights witch plate from a bedroom that your children slept in. Take the piece of door frame where your children's heights are still visible. If you love the birds singing while you sit on your deck, record the birdsong. A small jar of garden soil can be a memory of the beautiful flowers that were tended to. Take a leaf from the maple tree and place it in between the pages of a favourite book.

Of course, if you remove a piece of the house, fix and replace with a suitable, but neutral substitute so that no property damage results from your actions.

Break the Bad Memories

Whether from personal experience or though other's stories, we know that not all memories about a house are happy ones, just like not all of our experiences are positive ones. Sometimes change is good. An overall miserable existence in a certain house can be reason enough for someone to say "good riddens!" and have no desire to grieve the house. In fact, the feeling might be quite freeing, like an unburdening as the house is leaving your life.

You want to just leave the past behind and never look back.

One way to break the memories is to take a pottery bowl, a clay jar or even dinnerware, and simply break it to pieces. Smash it anyway you want. How you do it is irrelevant. What matters is the symbolic significance that the act of smashing that fragile object, holds. Break the negative energy and bad memories and move on with your life, never to return.

Another way is to go into the house and simply scream at it. Cry. Curse. Leave the pain and hurt there where it belongs. As you move on, it no longer belongs to you.

In the book "Carry Me Out Toes First", the author describes a real life emotional purging of a widow named Martha. Her anger over being left alone could no longer be contained and one night, her hell broke loose. It was only at the point where Martha acknowledged how the life she had, alone after her husband passed away, was the opposite of what she and her husband had talked about and planned for was she able to truly detach and move forward with her life.

Taking Care of Business

We all know what to do as we begin the process of emotional detachment from a home. The clearing, the cleaning, the decluttering and re-purposing. The making sure that every drawer and cupboard is gone through and is cleared out. Even the contents of the safety deposit box should be reviewed.

There is one piece of the journey that is a little strange to talk about, but it will be addressed here as it can be a very significant part of your experience. There is no judgement about the next suggestion, and it is simply a "heads up" to take care of what is in your personal life right now.

Let me tell you a story.

John (not his real name), was devastated after his wife passed away. She was healthy until the month before but a stroke took her from him very quickly. He was two years into his grieving and was finally seeing his way out of the sadness with the help of his faith and his large family.

His thoughts turned towards a possible move to the Canadian West Coast. He had travelled there several times after his wife passed, partly out of needing to escape from the loneliness of the large house and partly because he wanted to be closer to his youngest grandchildren. As it turned out, he liked the weather there much better than the prairies and decided to look at possibly selling the house that he and his wife owned since their first child was born, 45 years earlier.

He knew there was a safely deposit box, in his wife's name, at the local bank and had never thought to access it until now. The title to the house and all the paperwork was tucked away in it, so he thought.

The morning that John drove to the bank was warm and sunny and a perfect day…but why did it still feel strange to be thinking about selling the house without his wife? He missed her and wished they could be moving to the Coast together. He reached into his upper left hand shirt pocket to make sure the safety deposit box key was there, and smiled with a fleeting thought that the key was positioned over his heart.

The air conditioning in the bank kept the temperature comfortable, and John could not understand why he had a chill when he walked in. "Maybe I'm getting a cold", he thought to himself. The manager shook John's

The air conditioning in the bank kept the temperature comfortable, and John could not understand why he had a chill when he walked in. "Maybe I'm getting a cold", he thought to himself. The manager shook John's hand and they sat down at the counter as the signature card for the safety deposit box was presented for John's signature. There were only three other signatures on the card, all of them were his wife's. He looked at the date of her last signature. She last accessed the box nearly twenty years ago. He imagined her sitting here, at the same counter, writing her name on the card in that beautiful cursive font of hers. John shivered again from the blast of cold when the vault was open. He signed below his wife's entry. He was led to the box, and John slid the slender metal out of the casing, took it to the private area and closed the door behind him.

He sat on the plush blue padded chair and proceeded to open the box. The pastel pink title to the house was there, folded in half the long way, as well as the purchase contract from when they bought it and a yellowed, dog-eared drawing of the floor plan. A larger envelope contained photos of their wedding, which he thought was a little strange, and school photos of each of their 4 children at grade one. John held up a polaroid and felt a tear well up. The photo was of the entire family, John, the 4 children, and his wife, at a Christmas party when their youngest was still a baby. He thought how happy she looked back then. God, how he loved that woman.

He placed the title to the side of the safety deposit box. As he prepared to place the rest of the contents back in, he noticed a smaller brown envelope way in the back, almost out of sight.
His hand gently pried the folded brown envelope from the back of the metal box. As he straightened the fragile crease, he saw that his wife's name was written on the front of the envelope. The handwriting was angular and solid and he did not recognize it. He also noticed that the name on the envelope was his

wife's name before they were married.

John's heart skipped a beat.

John found a letter inside...

This story can unfold in any number of ways, but the main purpose is not to provide a solution to the mystery of the letter, nor is it to disclose the writer of it. The emotions that this story generates in you, the reader, is the pure intention. Each and every person will have a different response to this scenario and your response is your own experience. I wanted to open, in your own mind and heart, the emotional possibility of someone finding a very personal piece of your life when you are not around.

What needs to be taken care of right now before you even think about moving? Where are those precious intimate treasures hidden? Who would be devastated if they were found? Would the memory of you be turned upside down? The process of decluttering and clearing is not just about the china and books and clothing. Please remember that every drawer, every nook and cranny, from attic to basement will be cleared, and there may be something tucked away that you do NOT wish to see the light of day.

Where do YOU hide things? What things are deeply personal to you and to you alone? Do they need to be taken care of now? The time to take care of this task is while you are alive and are thinking clearly.

….and of course, whether or not it matters, is completely up to you…

Fur People

Our pets.

People who are not pet owners simply cannot grasp how important our furry companions are to us. In fact, people who are past the point of "needing" to move will stay tight and strong in their resolve to not displace their pet from the home. It is a true symbiotic relationship, as both the pet and the pet owner provide the other with love, nurturing and companionship. Sometimes the pet is one of the only living things that the homeowner sees for days on end and the connection is unbelievably strong.

If the pet passes, now the emotional journey of saying good bye to the house, becomes nearly impossible to bear. The one anchor, the one link to something living and real and the one relationship that has been unconditional and non-judgmental from the beginning, is gone. The grieving is not only for the loss of the best friend and faithful companion, but the home that housed them has now become painfully empty and quiet.

There are countless books and articles on the bond between humans and our fur people, but

the best way to understand is to talk with a pet owner, if you are not one yourself. I have heard stories where, if given an ultimatum, the pet owner will give up relationships with family before they give up on their pet.

If a move is absolutely necessary, people will not budge unless they can take their pet with them to the new home. Saying "goodbye house" to a house that is occupied by fur people is virtually impossible.

Moving in With Family

Relocating from your house can sometimes be made easier if family relationships support the option of living together. Now, even though this idea may send chills down the spines of most of us, there are fabulous examples of where this arrangement works beautifully.

Interestingly, most parts of the world do not have this problem. The multigenerational extended family all in one household IS the way most cultures of the world exist. The challenge that we in North America have, is that we all move out on our own, stressing "independence" and making it on our own as the flagship of success. If the idea of a "re-integration" of elder family members becomes a point of discussion, resistance is felt from both the children and the elder.

It appears as though this quirk is primarily a North American phenomenon, and will be further discussed in an upcoming publication exploring the dynamics of this cultural reality. Currently in production, the book "Senior Housing Options" will be a comprehensive overview of the choices in Alberta, and will provide some answers to the multitude of questions that adult children and the seniors themselves ask themselves throughout the journey of housing transition.

Does emotional journey of saying goodbye to your home exist in other counties? I don't have the answer to that one, but it sure does exist in Canada.
One local family found a solution that worked for them. As their mom's health declined, the family supported her in her own condo, and Ethel lived for many years as an elegant, beautifully independent elder. She had the "ouchies" of arthritis and "wheezies" of emphysema, but it was only when her macular degeneration rendered her nearly blind that Ethel's doctor suggested that she move to a lodge.

Ethel and her family had the type of relationship where things were always openly talked about in an atmosphere of respect. The children wanted to do the right thing by their Mom, and Ethel did not want to impose on her children. In fact, she was mortified to think that she would be putting her children out somehow if she were not in her own apartment. The emotional journey of this family totally revolved around love, and they came up with a plan that gave everyone respect and dignity.

Ethel accepted the invitation of her daughter and son-in-law to move in with them instead of into a care centre. Sean and Sheri had an extra bedroom in their bungalow villa along with its own bathroom and a walk-in shower. Sheri had a cat that was getting older, and she felt guilty leaving her fur-person at home alone all day while she went to work. Sean just wanted to do the right thing for his mother-in-law, as Ethel had always treated him kindly throughout the marriage to her daughter.

Yes, there really are still families like this!

The arrangement they came to was a fabulous one: instead of being in a care center, Ethel was with her own family and she and the pet kept each other company. Sean's job afforded him more flexibility with his time than Sheri's and he often was the person taking Ethel to her various appointments. Ethel did not like depending on anyone, even her family, so she made sure she at least contributed to the gas for the car and for the occasional dinner out with Sean and Sheri. Phone calls with her friends happened regularly and Ethel listened to audio books, since her eyesight was no longer good enough for her to read.

Luckily, Ethel "still has her noodles" and together, the family has openly talked about what would happen if this were not the case. Truth be told, there wasn't much discussion.

Ethel absolutely does not want to inconvenience her family and has given HER directions to her children, as well of having written copies of any documents at the lawyers.

Ethel, Sean and Sheri have taken the emotional goodbye of selling the apartment condo, and transformed the fear and angst into something that allows them all to have a richer, deeper connection.

The Business Part

The challenge of emotionally detaching from the home is not just happening with your family, it's a phenomenon that Brendon DeSimone, a real estate professional from San Francisco, California, has also witnessed. He has seen how the "love affair" that families have with their homes can actually work against them as they make decisions based on emotion rather than reason. His thought is that "what they're really doing is subconsciously sabotaging their chances for success, and that can cost them money in the end."

Acknowledge that selling your home can be stressful. Those who've been in their home just a few years are likely to have an easier time letting go than those who've lived there for decades or grew up in the house." His advice is to expect stress and emotion, and to not be surprised when those things show up for you. This will help you make better decisions down the road.

Make sure that you're ready to sell. Although it may seem obvious, he suggest that you "… take the time to ensure you're emotionally prepared for the sale. Talk to your agent and listen carefully to their suggestions. If you've

hired a competent agent and yet you're resisting their suggestions, that's a clue you may not be ready to let go. If so, don't sell just yet. Wait until you're ready."

He indicates that if you have no choice but to sell, it can be devastating emotionally, and to get as much support as you can from friends and family. Be honest with your agent about how difficult this is for you. Your agent is looking out for your best interests and acting on the assumption that you want to sell. If you're actually NOT ready to sell, the relationship is set to fail.

A final point Brendon makes is to "start thinking of your home as a product to be marketed". This is the most difficult realization for many families.

Quick Suggestions for Downsizing

Take a look at all the mail that comes to your home and begin to remove your address from mailing lists, cull the magazine subscriptions and reconsider the daily newspaper.

Start to get into the habit of removing two bags of recycling, old clothes or garbage for every one bag of anything that you bring into the house.

Discard the items that are "neutral", for example, expired coupons, old flyers, newspapers, community newsletters.

Now might be the time to begin using up your stockpiles of spices, laundry soap, toilet paper or anything else that you have around "just in case".

Stay away from any more bulk purchasing.

Re-purpose clothes that no longer fit or are no longer useful. How many pieces of clothing do you have that are just slightly imperfect with a broken zipper, a small stain on the front of a blouse, a torn seam? Consider either fixing them and wearing them, or simply repurpose.

Review all your old paper files one at a time: bank statements, bills, business cards, envelopes and greeting cards, etc.

It's ok to have an emotional attachment to the family home. It's ok to cry as you sort through your treasures.

Some Final Thoughts….

In closing, we can't make anyone do anything they don't want to do. All the logic in the world, all the reasoning in the world will not necessarily make someone change their mind. It is because the mind does the heart's bidding. Once the heart turns toward a choice, the mind is beckoned to follow. The heart guides the business part.

But if the heart is steadfast and solid in beating where it is, then all of the mind's cajoling, logic and fact will not move that heart. The mind does not control the heart.

Make no mistake: when given a choice, it is the heart that guides the business part. The heart guides your fingers as the pen places your signature on a contract. The most peaceful and most smooth transitions occur when the family's heart leads the way. There may still be pain and tears, but the angst is lessened. If humor and laughter can be mixed in, and an element of "feasting on your life", the emotional journey can be an opportunity for family to enjoy a moment where maybe, just maybe, their hearts can all beat together.

Marilyn Moldowan is a "Senior Real Estate Specialist" working out of Calgary, Alberta, Canada. Her consulting company is geared towards educating and guiding seniors and their families through their emotional journey as they begin the process of selling the family home. This preparation can take a year or more, but it can begin with small, step by step, concrete suggestions. The process is gentle and is based both in an understanding of the psychology of "home", and the heart centered way in which choices can be made. "Senior Condo Tours" is a service for people who choose to purchase an age appropriate condominium and is one way that the transition and facilitation between living styles can be accommodated. Her team includes hand-picked, seasoned, mature real estate professionals who are familiar with the emotional journey. They provide wisdom and compassion along with the business part of the sale of the home.

Marilyn Moldowan

"Senior Real Estate Specialist"....guiding the emotional journey of seniors and their families for four decades…

Thanks to the following contributors:

"They Left Us Everything"
by Plum Johnson

"The Art of Discarding: how to get rid of clutter and find joy" by Nagisa Tatsumi

"Carry Me Out Toes First"
by Marilyn Moldowan

"Recovering From Religion"
by Dendarah Hathorchuk

"The Upside of Your Dark Side"
by Todd Kashdan and Robert Biswas-Disner

Made in the USA
San Bernardino, CA
13 August 2017